My
Stupid
Headaches

MONTHLY TOTAL

MONTH

MONDAY	TUESDAY	WEDNESDAY	THURSDAY	FRIDAY	SATURDAY	SUNDAY

DATE

DURATION

INTENSITY

PAIN CHARACTERISTICS

TREATMENT

WHERE IT HURTS

FACTORS

SLEEP

CAFFEINE

ALCOHOL

WATER

FOOD

WEATHER

NOTES

OTHER FACTORS

DATE
DURATION
INTENSITY
PAIN CHARACTERISTICS
TREATMENT
WHERE IT HURTS
FACTORS
SLEEP
CAFFEINE
ALCOHOL
WATER
FOOD
WEATHER
NOTES
OTHER FACTORS

DATE

DURATION

INTENSITY

PAIN CHARACTERISTICS

TREATMENT

WHERE IT HURTS

FACTORS

SLEEP

CAFFEINE

ALCOHOL

WATER

FOOD

WEATHER

NOTES

OTHER FACTORS

DATE
DURATION
INTENSITY
PAIN CHARACTERISTICS
TREATMENT
WHERE IT HURTS
FACTORS
SLEEP
CAFFEINE
ALCOHOL
WATER
FOOD
WEATHER
NOTES
OTHER FACTORS

DATE
DURATION
INTENSITY
PAIN CHARACTERISTICS
TREATMENT
WHERE IT HURTS
FACTORS
SLEEP
CAFFEINE
ALCOHOL
WATER
FOOD
WEATHER
NOTES
OTHER FACTORS

DATE_______________________

DURATION_______________________

INTENSITY

PAIN CHARACTERISTICS

TREATMENT

WHERE IT HURTS

FACTORS

SLEEP

CAFFEINE

ALCOHOL

WATER

FOOD

WEATHER

NOTES

OTHER FACTORS

DATE_______________________   **DURATION**_______________

INTENSITY

PAIN CHARACTERISTICS

TREATMENT

WHERE IT HURTS

FACTORS

SLEEP

CAFFEINE

ALCOHOL

WATER

FOOD

WEATHER

OTHER FACTORS

NOTES

DATE
DURATION
INTENSITY
PAIN CHARACTERISTICS
TREATMENT
WHERE IT HURTS
FACTORS
SLEEP
OTHER FACTORS
CAFFEINE
ALCOHOL
WATER
FOOD
WEATHER
NOTES

DATE________________________

DURATION________________________

INTENSITY

PAIN CHARACTERISTICS

TREATMENT

WHERE IT HURTS

FACTORS

SLEEP

CAFFEINE

ALCOHOL

WATER

FOOD

WEATHER

NOTES

OTHER FACTORS

DATE

DURATION

INTENSITY

PAIN CHARACTERISTICS

TREATMENT

WHERE IT HURTS

FACTORS

SLEEP

CAFFEINE

ALCOHOL

WATER

FOOD

WEATHER

NOTES

OTHER FACTORS

DATE
DURATION
INTENSITY
PAIN CHARACTERISTICS
TREATMENT
WHERE IT HURTS
FACTORS
SLEEP
CAFFEINE
ALCOHOL
WATER
FOOD
WEATHER
NOTES
OTHER FACTORS

DATE___________________________

DURATION___________________________

INTENSITY

PAIN CHARACTERISTICS

TREATMENT

WHERE IT HURTS

FACTORS

SLEEP

CAFFEINE

ALCOHOL

WATER

FOOD

WEATHER

NOTES

OTHER FACTORS

DATE________________________

DURATION________________

INTENSITY

PAIN CHARACTERISTICS

TREATMENT

WHERE IT HURTS

FACTORS

SLEEP

CAFFEINE

ALCOHOL

WATER

FOOD

WEATHER

NOTES

OTHER FACTORS

DATE
DURATION
INTENSITY
PAIN CHARACTERISTICS
TREATMENT
WHERE IT HURTS
FACTORS
SLEEP
OTHER FACTORS
CAFFEINE
ALCOHOL
WATER
FOOD
WEATHER
NOTES

DATE
DURATION
WHERE IT HURTS
INTENSITY
PAIN CHARACTERISTICS
TREATMENT
FACTORS
SLEEP
OTHER FACTORS
CAFFEINE
ALCOHOL
WATER
FOOD
WEATHER
NOTES

DATE

DURATION

INTENSITY

PAIN CHARACTERISTICS

TREATMENT

WHERE IT HURTS

FACTORS

SLEEP

OTHER FACTORS

CAFFEINE

ALCOHOL

WATER

FOOD

WEATHER

NOTES

DATE
DURATION
INTENSITY
PAIN CHARACTERISTICS
TREATMENT
WHERE IT HURTS
FACTORS
SLEEP
CAFFEINE
ALCOHOL
WATER
FOOD
WEATHER
OTHER FACTORS
NOTES

DATE
DURATION
INTENSITY
PAIN CHARACTERISTICS
TREATMENT
WHERE IT HURTS
FACTORS
SLEEP
CAFFEINE
ALCOHOL
WATER
FOOD
WEATHER
NOTES
OTHER FACTORS

DATE_______________________

DURATION_______________________

INTENSITY

PAIN CHARACTERISTICS

TREATMENT

WHERE IT HURTS

FACTORS

SLEEP

CAFFEINE

ALCOHOL

WATER

FOOD

WEATHER

NOTES

OTHER FACTORS

DATE

DURATION

INTENSITY

PAIN CHARACTERISTICS

TREATMENT

WHERE IT HURTS

FACTORS

SLEEP

CAFFEINE

ALCOHOL

WATER

FOOD

WEATHER

NOTES

OTHER FACTORS

DATE

DURATION

INTENSITY

PAIN CHARACTERISTICS

TREATMENT

WHERE IT HURTS

FACTORS

SLEEP

CAFFEINE

ALCOHOL

WATER

FOOD

WEATHER

NOTES

OTHER FACTORS

DATE

DURATION

INTENSITY

PAIN CHARACTERISTICS

TREATMENT

FACTORS

SLEEP

CAFFEINE

ALCOHOL

WATER

FOOD

WEATHER

OTHER FACTORS

NOTES

DATE
DURATION
INTENSITY
PAIN CHARACTERISTICS
TREATMENT
WHERE IT HURTS
FACTORS
SLEEP
OTHER FACTORS
CAFFEINE
ALCOHOL
WATER
FOOD
WEATHER
NOTES

DATE________________________

DURATION________________________

INTENSITY

PAIN CHARACTERISTICS

TREATMENT

WHERE IT HURTS

FACTORS

SLEEP

CAFFEINE

ALCOHOL

WATER

FOOD

WEATHER

NOTES

OTHER FACTORS

DATE___________________________

DURATION___________________________

INTENSITY

PAIN CHARACTERISTICS

TREATMENT

WHERE IT HURTS

FACTORS

SLEEP

CAFFEINE

ALCOHOL

WATER

FOOD

WEATHER

NOTES

OTHER FACTORS

WHERE IT HURTS

INTENSITY

PAIN CHARACTERISTICS

TREATMENT

FACTORS

SLEEP

CAFFEINE

ALCOHOL

WATER

FOOD

WEATHER

NOTES

OTHER FACTORS

DATE
DURATION
INTENSITY
PAIN CHARACTERISTICS
TREATMENT
WHERE IT HURTS
FACTORS
SLEEP
OTHER FACTORS
CAFFEINE
ALCOHOL
WATER
FOOD
WEATHER
NOTES

WHERE IT HURTS

FACTORS

SLEEP

CAFFEINE

ALCOHOL

WATER

FOOD

WEATHER

NOTES

OTHER FACTORS

FACTORS

SLEEP

CAFFEINE

ALCOHOL

WATER

FOOD

WEATHER

NOTES

OTHER FACTORS

DATE___________________

DURATION___________________

INTENSITY

PAIN CHARACTERISTICS

TREATMENT

WHERE IT HURTS

FACTORS

SLEEP

CAFFEINE

ALCOHOL

WATER

FOOD

WEATHER

NOTES

OTHER FACTORS

DATE________________________

DURATION________________________

INTENSITY

PAIN CHARACTERISTICS

TREATMENT

WHERE IT HURTS

FACTORS

SLEEP

CAFFEINE

ALCOHOL

WATER

FOOD

WEATHER

OTHER FACTORS

NOTES

DATE

DURATION

INTENSITY

PAIN CHARACTERISTICS

TREATMENT

WHERE IT HURTS

FACTORS

SLEEP

CAFFEINE

ALCOHOL

WATER

FOOD

WEATHER

OTHER FACTORS

NOTES

DATE

DURATION

INTENSITY

PAIN CHARACTERISTICS

TREATMENT

WHERE IT HURTS

FACTORS

SLEEP

CAFFEINE

ALCOHOL

WATER

FOOD

WEATHER

OTHER FACTORS

NOTES

DATE_______________________

DURATION_______________________

INTENSITY

PAIN CHARACTERISTICS

TREATMENT

WHERE IT HURTS

FACTORS

SLEEP

CAFFEINE

ALCOHOL

WATER

FOOD

WEATHER

NOTES

OTHER FACTORS

DATE___________________ **DURATION**___________________

INTENSITY

PAIN CHARACTERISTICS

TREATMENT

WHERE IT HURTS

FACTORS

SLEEP   OTHER FACTORS

CAFFEINE

ALCOHOL

WATER

FOOD

WEATHER

NOTES

DATE____________________
DURATION____________________
WHERE IT HURTS
INTENSITY
PAIN CHARACTERISTICS
TREATMENT
FACTORS
SLEEP
CAFFEINE
ALCOHOL
WATER
FOOD
WEATHER
OTHER FACTORS
NOTES

DATE_____________________

DURATION_____________________

WHERE IT HURTS

INTENSITY

PAIN CHARACTERISTICS

TREATMENT

FACTORS

SLEEP

CAFFEINE

ALCOHOL

WATER

FOOD

WEATHER

OTHER FACTORS

NOTES

FACTORS

SLEEP

CAFFEINE

ALCOHOL

WATER

FOOD

WEATHER

NOTES

OTHER FACTORS

DATE________________________

DURATION________________________

INTENSITY

PAIN CHARACTERISTICS

TREATMENT

WHERE IT HURTS

FACTORS

SLEEP

CAFFEINE

ALCOHOL

WATER

FOOD

WEATHER

NOTES

OTHER FACTORS

INTENSITY

PAIN CHARACTERISTICS

TREATMENT

FACTORS

SLEEP

CAFFEINE

ALCOHOL

WATER

FOOD

WEATHER

NOTES

OTHER FACTORS

DATE______________________________

DURATION____________________

INTENSITY

PAIN CHARACTERISTICS

TREATMENT

WHERE IT HURTS

FACTORS

SLEEP

CAFFEINE

ALCOHOL

WATER

FOOD

WEATHER

OTHER FACTORS

NOTES

DATE______________________

DURATION______________________

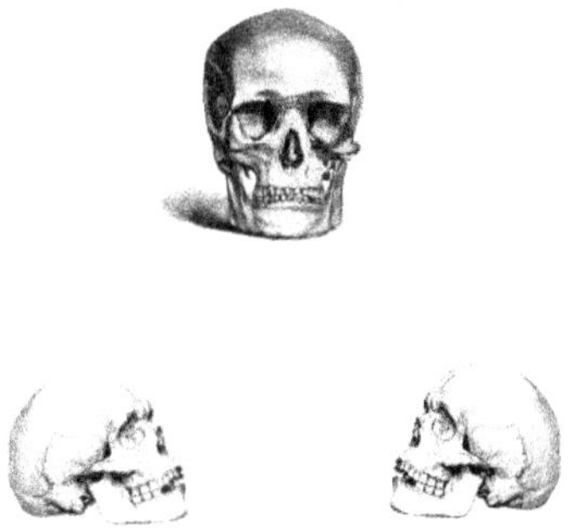

WHERE IT HURTS

INTENSITY

PAIN CHARACTERISTICS

TREATMENT

FACTORS

SLEEP

CAFFEINE

ALCOHOL

WATER

FOOD

WEATHER

OTHER FACTORS

NOTES

DATE
DURATION
INTENSITY
PAIN CHARACTERISTICS
TREATMENT
WHERE IT HURTS
FACTORS
SLEEP
CAFFEINE
ALCOHOL
WATER
FOOD
WEATHER
NOTES
OTHER FACTORS

FACTORS

SLEEP

OTHER FACTORS

CAFFEINE

ALCOHOL

WATER

FOOD

WEATHER

NOTES

DATE________________________

DURATION________________________

INTENSITY

PAIN CHARACTERISTICS

TREATMENT

WHERE IT HURTS

FACTORS

SLEEP

CAFFEINE

ALCOHOL

WATER

FOOD

WEATHER

OTHER FACTORS

NOTES

DATE_________________________________

DURATION_____________________________

WHERE IT HURTS

INTENSITY

PAIN CHARACTERISTICS

TREATMENT

FACTORS

SLEEP

CAFFEINE

ALCOHOL

WATER

FOOD

WEATHER

NOTES

OTHER FACTORS

DATE
DURATION
INTENSITY
PAIN CHARACTERISTICS
TREATMENT
WHERE IT HURTS
FACTORS
SLEEP
OTHER FACTORS
CAFFEINE
ALCOHOL
WATER
FOOD
WEATHER
NOTES

DATE_________________________
DURATION_____________________

INTENSITY

PAIN CHARACTERISTICS

TREATMENT

WHERE IT HURTS

FACTORS

SLEEP

CAFFEINE

ALCOHOL

WATER

FOOD

WEATHER

NOTES

OTHER FACTORS